WAKE UP AND UNLEASH YOUR UNLIMITED POWER NOW

REAL LIFE CALISTHENICS STORY

Todor Djordjevic

TABLE OF CONTENTS

MOTTO

"My inner-motivation and self-discipline techniques are based on Napoleon Hill's and Arnold Schwarzenegger's Principles of Success. I don't believe in limits and plateaus. They are only created by our mind. I believe in persistence, patience, productivity, and possibility. These qualities always produce results!"

ABOUT THE AUTHOR

Todor Djordjevic is a 46-year-old Yugoslavian-American founder of Tosha Fitness. He is an award winner for the most diverse fitness and education world perspective. He is an athlete, international fitness and health expert, cross-cultural specialist, and a real-estate investor.

He has entered the global stage with the book 10 Super Easy Steps to Your Dream Body 3x. In particular, his 3x Body Fat Attack Program has helped many to become physically fit.

He worked with the U.S. Department of State as an educator in South-East Asia, the Arabic Gulf and the U.S.A. He has also written fitness articles for Serbian Men's Health and Fitness Magazine.

Please refer to the following links about Todor:

Http://www.toshafitness.com

Http://www.menshealth.rs/fitness/6264

http://www.menshealth.rs/fitness/2931

INTRODUCTION

I want to thank you and congratulate you for downloading the book, *"Wake Up and Unleash Your Unlimited Power Now: Real Life Calisthenics Story"*.

Are you trying to get in shape but hate going to your local gym? Do you want to be more flexible and leaner; not just skinny-fat? Do you want to enjoy your time outdoors, and have more fun when you exercise?

The best of all, what if there's a way through which you can achieve your fitness goals without paying expensive gym membership fees? How about losing your belly fat and increasing your muscle mass gradually with creative exercises?

Do you want to train smart, be more positive, and have tons of fun?

That would be just amazing, right?

Well, in this book, you will learn that whatever you do today will truly matter tomorrow.

This book contains valuable information that will help you increase your inner-motivation and activate your true strength, so you can get the body you have always wanted.

In this book, you'll learn the following: how to think like a champion, succeed while failing, be persistent towards your goal, and train smart, which in turn, will help you lose those excess pounds and eventually maintain your ideal weight.

Thanks again for downloading this book, I hope you enjoy it!

CHAPTER 1

DON'T BE LIKE EVERYONE ELSE

There is Unlimited Power Within You!

The power that runs through your veins is like a fountain of endless youth that never runs out of water. It is like a beautiful white swan who always swims at your favorite lake.

There is something so strong and unique within you, that it could move mountains, transform people, and create world peace. In addition, this inner-power could shape your personality and enlighten you in most difficult moments. It could also help you to act righteously and achieve all your dream goals. It becomes your most powerful weapon when you definitely need it. It has always been a part of you, and it truly defines you. What is it?

It is the Power of Your Decision.

If you are like everyone else, you might be full of excuses, like to do things the easy way, and have a couple of extra pounds. You might always wait for the right moment to start something new. Then, when you finally start, after the first difficulty, you might easily quit. You most likely do not start again the same thing, as you have previously failed. Then, the endless cycle of starting and quitting goes on and on. This way you not just fail, but you are a failure. Do you want to be like that?

Remember that your life is full of unlimited possibilities. Elite athletes once have made their decision to start training seriously. And, they trained like their life depended on it. They never gave up on their way to success. They were persistent to move forward and become the best. They became champions because of the power of their decision to take an immediate action.

For example, Pele, the greatest soccer player of all time, grew up in the poverty of crime ridden ghetto of Sao Paolo. His strong inner-motivation to play soccer was his key to success. He had truly inspired and touched hearts of millions, not just in his own country; but all over the world.

If Arnold Schwarzenegger had never stepped outside of his comfort zone, he would still be a yearling in the Austrian Alps. He said: "Break the rules not the law."

Think for a second and ask yourself who you want to be and how badly you want success. What are you waiting for?

Calisthenics Loves You!

I love calisthenics. How about you? I bet you might not even know what it is.

***URBAN CALISTHENICS** or simply known as **CALISTHENICS** are a Street Workout that involves physical activity performed mostly in outdoor parks or public facilities.*

I describe it as a form of modern gymnastics with free movements through space that include, but are not limited to: pulling or pushing oneself up, bending, jumping, or swinging. Body-weight is constantly used for resistance in order to improve someone's agility, balance, and coordination.

For four decades, and I literally mean it, I was clueless about calisthenics. I was drawn into playing tennis, swimming, and working-out indoors, instead. I remember practicing my tennis serve for hours with my dad, and then swimming at the local lake. I had also spent endless hours at the gym with some mixed results.

In July 2018, for the very first time, I accidentally watched a YouTube video called a Park Hour. There was a college student bar-spinning outside in the park. Fitness motivational music was accompanying the video. I thought, wow very cool. How could I do the same?

Everything on that video looked very impressive and relatively easy to do. I was sure that something "too easy" required heavy work to make it perfect. Later, the same video brought a fresh perspective to my calisthenics beginning. It simply motivated me to try something new.

CHAPTER 2
THE GAME OF LIFE

Work Hard or Hardly Work?
It is most likely that people blessed with a pleasant climate year around prefer outdoor activities. Alternatively, people in hot climates would convince you the opposite. They might tell you that indoor activities are their favorite.

One thing I know for sure is that everyone is right in their own eyes. We all have different points of view, different hobbies, and interests that truly shape our individua. One thing we all have in similarity are our excuses. They always sound the same wherever we go.

No matter of your physical activity preference and location, doctors all over the world agree about the same thing. The physical activity is necessary for one's well-being. So then, why are we still sedentary and inactive?

Be physically active and persistent in order to achieve your fitness goals. You are either your biggest enemy or your best friend. Whatever you plant in your mind will either grow a poisonous weed or a beautiful flower.

Each of us leaves either positive, neutral, or negative impressions on someone else. You have probably heard the saying that your success is closely related to what your best friends do. In other words, if the people who surround you are negative, you might the be the same. Alternatively, if they are optimistic and hardworking, you will be too.

Negative people should not be a part of your life. If it is work related then tolerate them, show respect, and try to avoid conflict. On the other hand, people that repeatedly leave positive impressions on you are the ones who could inspire you to excel in the field of your choice. Be smart and carefully choose your friends.

Success Means Failing Over Again and Again

Remember that smart people are not afraid to experiment to try something new. They fail a multiple number of times on their way to success, but they never give up. They stand firm and try again. They learn from their own mistakes. Finally, they succeed because they run out of all failure. On the other hand, there are others who allow circumstances to shape their future. Are you one of them?

We all play the same game of life. In this game, no one truly wins. Some of us move fast forward and achieve their goals, while others simply stay behind.

When we are young, we rarely think about our time. We always have plenty of time to do anything. Our parents usually dictate our daily chores. We do what we are told. We do not question or overthink. Everything goes smoothly and in control.

As adults, we see our time really passing fast. We become more aware of our surroundings. We realize that we have different choices in life. Some of us work hard, the other ones hardly work.

We measure the time in seconds, minutes, hours, days, months, and years. Before we are even aware of it, there is a new day, a new month, or a new year. How many times have you wished you would have completed something earlier? Are you endlessly waiting for the right moment to start something new that truly matters?

You Are a Super-Star

Are we too busy, or just too full of excuses? One day all over the world has the same 24 hours. If the clock's hand always moves forward, why do we not do the same?

Your mom has probably told you not to start tomorrow something you could finish today. What is that it truly matters to you? What is that you cannot live without? What drives you out of bed every morning? Don't wait until tomorrow to compete something you could finish today. It might be too late!

We become what we think about most of the time. If you believe that you are a great French-Horn player, and you put an extra effort to practice playing this instrument daily, you will become one.

As a twelve-year-old kid, I didn't mind practicing a French-Horn after school hours. I believed I must be disciplined and work hard to become a famous musician. Four years later, my persistence and soldier-like discipline finally paid off. I was the best French-Horn player in Yugoslavia. I played multiple times on national TV and even had my own LP record.

God always opens new doors to those who believe and work hard towards their goals. Don't forget to knock at the door first. Then, work hard on your future goals and believe it is possible. God will open any door for you. He wants you to succeed in anything you dreamed about. Remember, you should always make a first step forward!

Every morning when you wake up repeat ten times: "Something good is going to happen to me today!" Give gratitude to God and just watch for the miracle to happen. No matter how busy you are, or how happy or disappointing your life might be, giving gratitude to God should always be your priority.

Remember God is the one who wants you to succeed. He is the one who makes you a super-star. So, acknowledge him in anything you do in realization of your dream goals.

Two Steps Forward, One Step Back

Confucius ones said: "It is not important how slowly we are moving forward if we are progressing towards realization of our future goals."

The road to success is not simple. It is not a straight line, as well. It might require that you learn a new skill or put an extra effort in order to succeed.

If you are achieving your future goals, one step behind does not truly matter. A challenging situation might provide a valuable experience, while success creates unforgettable memories. It is inevitable you will learn to overcome obstacles on your road to success.

Don't worry if your road to success is less travelled. You are not the only one suffering. The difference between you and the others is that you have a feasible goal, and they might not. Instead of complaining, be sure you are constantly moving forward. How slowly you go on this road less travelled is simply not important. It is crucial that you never stop moving forward.

Remember that a person without a goal is lost. And, one who is not progressing in the field of his choice is wasted. Try to do the things the hard way instead and watch yourself grow. Learn from your own mistakes on your way to success. Tell yourself: "Just do it!" Then, take an immediate action, and you will succeed.

Finally, do not be another Mr. and Mrs. Excuse. The world today is already full of people who do everything the easy way. They are literally anywhere and everywhere.

CHAPTER 3
NO GYM, NO DIET... NO PROBLEM

Determine Your Fitness Goals First

Before you start your workout, make sure your goals are concise and clear. You might want to improve your strength, flexibility, or core. Do you want to become faster or leaner? Whatever your goals are, try to choose something you enjoy. Do not proceed with something you were pushed to do, unless you are convinced you will succeed. Also, be aware if you are training just to impress someone, you might tremble and fall.

The main reason people do not achieve their fitness goals is because they don't try hard enough. They might not have a right attitude to succeed. Their goals might be vague, and their progress limited. Bruce Lee once said: "I don't believe in limits in anything I do. I go beyond plateaus on my way to success."

Try to copy the attitude of successful people in order to achieve all your dream goals. Pick up their positive vibes, at first. Next, fully immerse yourself in their minds. Then, think and act the way they do. Mirror and follow their activities, and fully observe their reactions. Finally, watch yourself grow tremendously on your way to success.

The Dieters and The Gym Rats are Wrong

What would happen to you if you just follow a diet regimen and lose weight? Yes, you will become slimmer after a couple of weeks. Yes, you will look leaner. But, in reality, are you going to be any stronger? Are you going to have those chiseled well-toned muscles? Honestly, it is very likely you will lose your muscle mass without exercise. In addition, you will become weaker then you were before. That is why this is not a right option for you.

Dieters appear slimmer, they might look better in the mirror than before, but their yo-yo diet will take havoc on their metabolism, and if their daily calories fell more than recommended daily calories for men and women, they will jeopardize their own health. Most people belong to this category even though they don't even realize it. People are trying to find shortcuts in health. Unfortunately, once people destroy their own health, it is very difficult to get it back.

Gym enthusiasts somehow falsely believe in amazing fitness and health benefits of lifting weights. I don't doubt the gym helps them to gain necessary strength and increased muscle mass. In addition, their overall health could improve, as well. But, that's about it. What happens to their flexibility? Are there just getting bulkier or more flexible and stronger? Is their core any stronger?

It is most likely that no one, except gymnasts and people in calisthenics, could spin on the high-bar without the adequate training. The gym rats' flexibility has always been an issue. Their core muscles are usually their weak point, as well. Lifting weights is often associated to increased bulkiness, but decreased flexibility. One thing we know for sure is that pumping iron could help you increase your strength. For most of the men this is good enough. Are you one of them?

By taking illegal supplements millions destroy their health fast. Liver and kidneys are the first ones to suffer from illegal supplement abuse. Then, heart problems follow. At the end, one's overall health is fully destroyed and could not be brought back.

On the other hand, if proper exercises are implemented, the body weight exercises could be a solution to many health problems. Unfortunately, pumping iron at the gym cannot solve all ailments, but can help you stay healthy.

CHAPTER 4
THE TRUE STRENGTH LIES HERE

Calisthenics Rock

The true strength comes from performing calisthenics; or how they call it a street workout.

When gymnastics is performed outdoors in the park it becomes calisthenics. On You Tube you might find the calisthenics under the following names: the park hour, street workout, or bar calisthenics, etc.

Here is why I have completely switched my indoor gym hours with sunshine-calisthenics park-hour. In my point of view, there are three major reasons why calisthenics rock:

1. Outdoor calisthenics increases vitamin D levels necessary for T production. Also, the hormones of happiness known as endorphins are fully developed during a 45-minute medium intensity outdoor workout.

2. True core strength is developed with outdoor calisthenics. Various compound body exercises activate large groups of muscles at the same time and positively contribute to one's core strength. For example, L seat, V seat, dragon flag, or front and back lever could help you develop a six-pack much faster than the regular indoor gym.

3. Outdoor calisthenics help one to complete a full body workout every time. It is truly fantastic that most of the muscles are trained at the same time. The exercises are often complex and might require isolation exercise training before they are fully executed.

Warm Up First

Complex compound exercises should never be performed without a proper warm-up. Single, isolated, muscle groups need to be activated first in order to complete more complex movements.

For example, spinning on the high-bar has the following prerequisites:

    a. A variety of pull-ups, dips, and push-ups need to be completed first in order to improve your arm strength.

    b. L-seat with half and full extended legs is necessary in order to improve core muscle strength. In addition, V-seat could be added during L-seat practice, by pulling the legs straight up for a couple of seconds in order to create tension.

    c. Standing one-leg hand-toe touch could be performed during warm up to improve overall flexibility.

Calisthenics Fit for Life

Remember that cavemen were fit, not only because of what they ate, but because of their physical activity. A nice thing about calisthenics is that you don't need to go to the gym to get fit. You also don't need to climb the trees or to hunt wild animals for survival. All you need to do is to locate the calisthenics park in your neighborhood and put a bit effort to learn something new. Calisthenics exercises are creative and fun.

Calisthenics will help you lose weight and increase muscle mass naturally with maximum results. You will think positively and develop inner-motivation to achieve not just your fitness goals, but also any other goals. At the end, you will not just have a good time outdoors, but you will stay fit the rest of your life. So, what are you waiting for? Just do it!

SPINNING ON THE HIGH-CROOKED-BAR

REAL LIFE CALISTHENICS STORY

ABOUT THE HIGH-CROOKED-BAR

There was this crooked calisthenics high-bar proudly aging disgracefully in the calisthenics park. A poor construction had the high-bar on one side standing at 6 feet tall, while the other side was at 6.2 feet above the ground. A whole construction had a shaky base with a cracked cement around it.

No one really cared about the poor bar. No one even liked it. And of course, whoever said there was a reason, it was right. The gypsies have even tried unsuccessfully to destroy the bar completely and sell it for recycled iron.

DA THING OF MA-GIC

A half broken, twisted, vertical metal rod was the bar's construction main decoration for years. The poor 'thing of ma- gic' was also so seriously shaking when in use, that literally no one dare to use it. A whole construction was on the edge of collapse, and it just waited for it right time to fully give up.

The upper bar of 'da thing of ma-gic' was built so high that one had to seriously jump first and then do the pull-up, in order to spin over the bar. Finally, while one being on the top of the high-bar, a whole construction would start shaking enough to remind you of how much she hated you.

There were months and months I had spent in heavy basic calisthenics training while improving my strength, flexibility, and the core. I had completed more than 1000s of pull-ups, push-ups etc. before I ever first approached the cruel high-bar.

I remember succeeding performing a pull-over on a nearby 5.7 feet bar first. Somehow, the evil 6.2 feet high-bar was not my style, so I had fully ignored it.

SPINNING ON THE HIGH-CROOKED-BAR DETAILS

ABOUT MR. X

One fine day, after more than three months of heavy outdoor- calisthenics-basic-training, everything changed. There was this guy whose name I don't know (I will call him "Mr. X,) who came to the park and changed my whole calisthenics perspective.

Mr. X had an intention to conquer the evil high-bar and spin over it. The problem with him was that he had never conquered a lower 5.7 feet bar first. Everyone normal would tell him to conquer the lower bar first (which was next to the 6.2 feet bar) before he moves to the higher elevation bar.

Mr. X was in his early 30s constantly failing in performing a high-bar spin on the 6.2 feet bar. He was not a gymnast nor a gym rat. He was just a regular guy who wanted to conquer the evil bar.

While being asked why he was not practicing on the nearby 5.7 feet bar, Mr. X said that he wanted to conquer the 6.2

feet bar first. The guy was so persistent, that for months I could not convince him to practice on the lower bar first.

He was so persistent in training on the high-bar that one day he was training with his sprained ankle. He said that he was practicing this move from 2009. And now we were deeply at the end of 2018.

Day by day, for more than a month, I was training on the 5.7 feet bar. I pointed out that Mr. X needed to train on this lower bar first to develop necessary strength for a spin on a higher 6.2 fee bar. I have showed him the necessary variety of pull-ups and other basic-calisthenics exercises that he needed first to gain the necessary strength.

THE GREAT SURPRISE

Finally, no one could stop Mr. X from his crazy idea to conquer the 6.2 feet bar. After seeing him fail to complete a full high-bar spin day by day, nor being able to convince him to practice on a lower 5.7 feet bar, I have decided to try the following new method.

I went straight to the 6.2 feet bar and turned the video recording mode on my digital camera. After 3 months of heavy training, for the very first time, I had greatly surprised myself. I was able to do two complete pull-over spins on the evil 6.2 feet high-bar. Mr. X, who was watching me, had just stayed speechless. I caught this amazing moment on the camera, and immediately embedded it on the YouTube as the recorded proof.

Here is the YouTube link:

https://youtu.be/99RHiKkY68M

GOD IS ALMIGHTY

At the very end, I was really proud to motivate Mr. X to keep training and to never give up. His dream of pulling-over the 6.2 feet bar is still in progress. Just recently, he has succeeded hanging on that high bar with both of his knees, which is more than half work being done.

My dream to conquer a high-crooked-bar is reality. Nowadays, whenever I work out in the park, first I must spin over the same crooked bar in order to prove that my dream is still alive.

I must admit that Mr. X and his crazy endless efforts greatly inspired me to perform at my best and conquer the difficult crooked high-bar spin. I was able to defeat the failure. I was able to win the battle against myself. I was able to redefine impossible to I'm Possible.

God has helped me to shine like a star. God is almighty.

Thank you, God, for your guidance and unlimited support.

Conclusion

Thank you again for downloading this book!

I hope this book has provided a step forward towards your new healthier body. Your decision today to give a chance to calisthenics could mean fit for the rest of your life for you.

The next step is to implement what you have learned. Locate the calisthenics park in your neighborhood and exercise. Make sure you work steadily towards your fitness goals. Be a patient, hardworking optimist.

Remember that health is your wealth. This is cliché, but it is true. You can't enjoy life if conditions burden you such as diabetes or hypertension. Live a healthier, fuller, and happier life by exercising daily.

Finally, if you enjoyed this book, please take the time to share your thoughts and post a review on Amazon. It'd be greatly appreciated.

Check Out My Other Books

Below you'll find some of my other books that are popular on Amazon and Kindle as well. Simply click on the links below to check them out. Alternatively, you can visit http://www.toshafitness.com to see other work done by me.

http://amzn.to/1UlMKRM - This is My Other Book on Amazon

http://amzn.to/1tzWMXB - This is My Other Book on Amazon

http://amzn.to/2baLpR9 - This is My Other Book on Amazon

http://amzn.to/1RNhiy9 - This Is My Other Book on Amazon

http://amzn.to/1nTeVvC - This is My Other Book on Amazon

If the links do not work, for whatever reason, you can simply search for these titles on the Amazon website to find them.

Bonus

Subscribe to Tosha Fitness Newsletter

By subscribing to Tosha Fitness Newsletter at http://www.toshafitness.com you will get free access to the newest fitness and diet trends and tips. At the same time, I have included a completely free Pdf report from one of my bestselling books on Amazon.
Remember that your goal is to be better than you were yesterday. Keep moving forward and believe in yourself. Your dreams are possible.

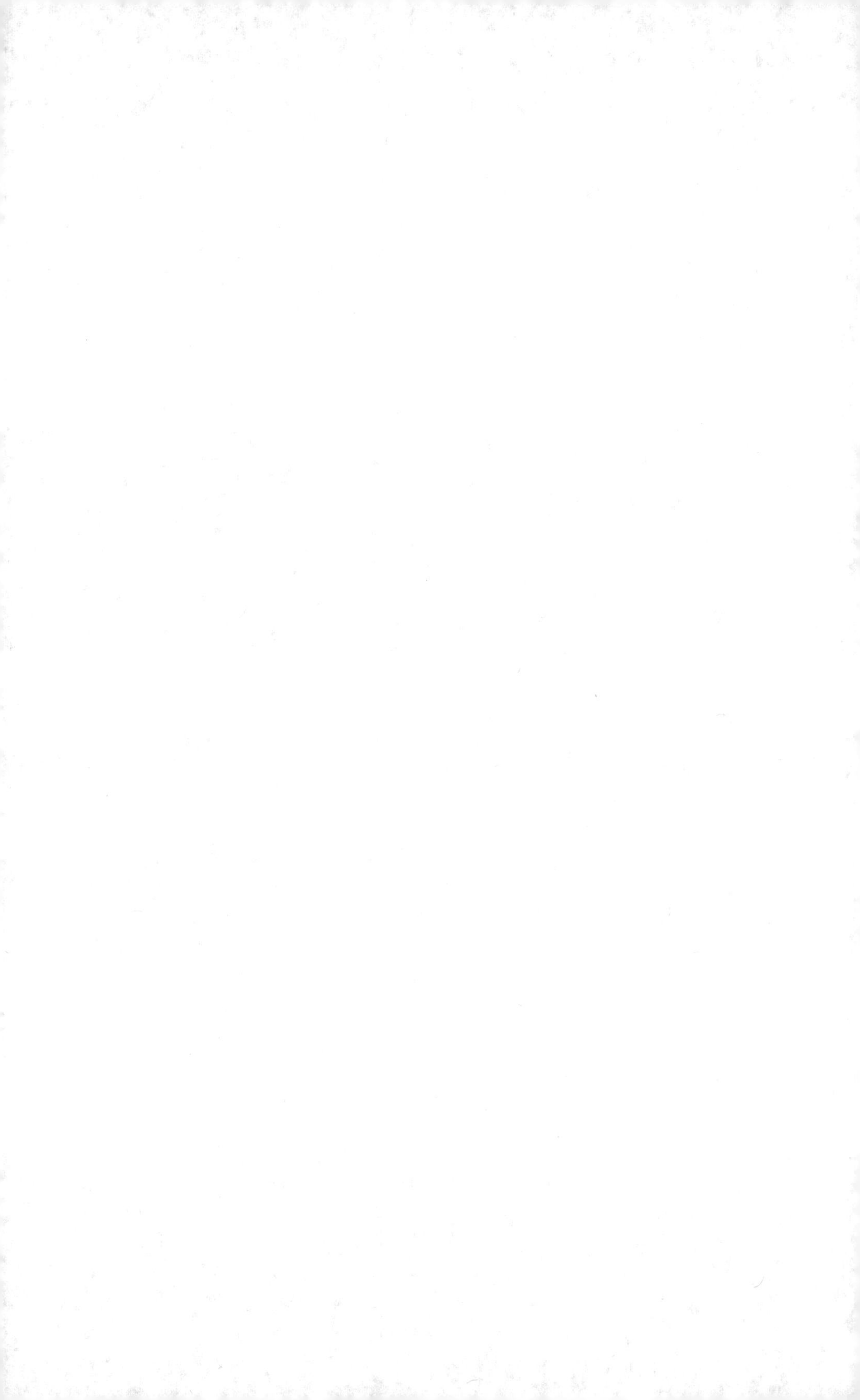

9 781731 059277